50 Ways to Sleep Better

In Association with
The Sleep Disorders Center
Columbia-Presbyterian Medical Center

Neil B. Kavey, M.D.

D1496702

Contributors:

The Sleep Disorders Center at Columbia-Presbyterian Medical Center is a highly specialized outpatient facility for the evaluation and treatment of patients with problems related to sleep and wakefulness. Established in 1977, The Sleep Disorders Center was among the first centers in the United States devoted exclusively to the practice of sleep disorder medicine. The Center's staff integrated the knowledge of sleep and wakefulness obtained from a variety of medical and academic sources.

Neil B. Kavey, M.D., is the director of The Sleep Disorders Center at Columbia-Presbyterian Medical Center. He also holds a position on the Board of Directors for the American Sleep Disorders Association and is a member of the Sleep Research Society. He has conducted extensive research and authored many publications in the area of sleep disorder medicine.

Cover Photo: Chris Harvey/Tony Stone Images

CONTENTS

CONTENTS

HELPING CHILDREN SLEEP BETTER

50 WAYS TO SLEEP BETTER

INTRODUCTION

Knowledge about sleep and sleep disorders is one of the final frontiers in the study of human biology. Although we spend approximately one third of our lives asleep, until recently there was little scientific study of sleep and no knowledge at all of sleep disorders.

The big breakthrough in our understanding of sleep did not come until 1957 when scientists discovered there actually are two different kinds of sleep. One type, rapid eye movement (REM) sleep, is named for the distinctive shifting of the eyes that occurs. Dreaming is almost entirely limited to REM sleep. During REM sleep, the muscles are paralyzed and the body, virtually motionless. The brain, however, is just as active as it is when you are awake. The second type is termed non-REM sleep, during which rapid eye movements are absent. Non-REM sleep is often very deep, involving both mental and physical inactivity.

The discovery of REM sleep and non-REM sleep caused great excitement among scientists. Research into sleep was conducted with newfound energy. Most work was directed toward learning about normal sleep, but discoveries were made concerning abnormal sleep. In this fashion the science of sleep disorders was created.

Before long the field of sleep disorders moved from the laboratory into the physician's office. Experts in abnormal sleep applied their efforts to the acquisition of knowledge and to the diagnosis and treatment of sleep disorders. Medical facilities devoted exclusively to sleep were established. With the creation of these sleep centers, people with problems related to sleep and wakefulness had a place to turn for advice, diagnosis, and treatment of their symptoms.

This book represents, in part, the results of the past 37 years of sleep research and clinical practice of sleep medicine—the combined experience of thousands of scientists and physicians. It contains 50 tips and techniques that will help you sleep soundly through the night and be alert and awake throughout the entire day.

The book is divided into five sections. Section One deals with the primary sleep disorders—conditions that almost always require medical attention. The focus is on recognizing when a real medical problem exists and where to turn for help. Some of the most common disorders are discussed in detail.

Section Two is devoted to measures you can take during the day to improve sleep quality. We all recognize that sleep at night affects how we feel during the day. Less obvious is that what we do during the day affects the way we sleep at night. This group of tips is directed toward modifying daytime behavior in an attempt to ensure sound, restful sleep.

Section Three discusses aspects of the sleep-wake schedule that impact sleep quality. The invention of the electric light changed our work and recreation schedules and thus our sleep schedules. The result is often poor sleep. Shift work and jet lag, two sleep problems that were virtually unknown until this century, are among those mentioned here.

Section Four addresses issues related to the sleep environment, that is, the setting in which sleep occurs. Every aspect of the bedroom from the temperature in the room to the firmness of the mattress can affect sleep quality. The remedies in this section identify specific problems related to the sleep environment and discuss how to correct them.

The final section is devoted entirely to the special sleep problems of children. A child's sleep is important to his or her growth and development, but a child's sleeping problem inevitably affects the sleep of the entire family. Successfully dealing with problems that are specific to childhood helps ensure that everyone in the household obtains a good night's sleep.

If you would like further information about sleep or sleep disorders, call or write: National Sleep Foundation, 122 South Robertson Blvd., Suite 201, Los Angeles, CA 90048, (310) 288-0466.

Alternatively, you can contact your local sleep disorders center. For the location of the nearest sleep center, call or write: American Sleep Disorders Association, 1610 14th Street Northwest, Suite 300, Rochester, MN 55901, (507) 287-6006.

1

KNOW HOW MUCH IS ENOUGH.

You've come home from work, had a bite to eat, and settled in. Your plan is to watch the news and as much of David Letterman's antics as you can before you fall asleep. But while you're putting on your pajamas, your roommate is dressing to meet a friend at a local club. The two of you start work at the same time! Night after night she's just getting started while you're winding down. And morning after morning, she's out of bed at about the same time you are. How does she do it? And why can't you?

Does this scenario sound familiar? First, you should know the habits of each of these people are perfectly normal. Our need for sleep is as individual as we are. Although most of us need between six and nine hours a night (most of us sleep about 7.5 hours a night), others may require far more—or less. Those at the extreme ends of the sleeping spectrum are called "long sleepers" or "short sleepers."

Long sleepers can take a lot of flack for the number of hours they sleep, but these people are not lazy or poorly motivated. They simply need more sleep. And if you're one of those people who feels there just aren't enough hours in a day, you may admire short sleepers for their ability to stay awake. But as the second sample scenario demonstrates, they may find the hours alone when everyone else is asleep unsettling. Short sleepers often believe they have insomnia, when in fact they feel well rested after just a few hours of sleep.

Here are a few tips to help you stop losing sleep over the number of winks you need.

For short sleepers

- Stop worrying. Sleeping five or fewer hours a day isn't harmful if that's all your body needs.

- Use the time well. View the extra hours of wakefulness as an opportunity for productive work, recreation, or relaxation.

For long sleepers

- Budget sleep time. Accept the fact that you need lots of sleep, and fit that time into your daily schedule. You may actually accomplish more if you allow yourself the extra time to sleep because you'll be well rested!

- Ignore any negative comments about your sleep needs. Don't let other people's opinions affect you. You're not getting "too much sleep." You're getting what you need.

For everyone

- There is no "right" number of hours for sleep. Each of us has our own sleep needs.

- Listen to your body. It'll tell you if you're getting enough sleep. If you feel well rested and alert for most or all of the day, your total sleep time is adequate. But if you're tired or dragging for much of the day, you may need to get more sleep—even if you're getting eight hours.

- Know how much sleep your body needs and accept it. You may have to adapt your lifestyle a bit to accommodate your sleep needs, but you'll be more alert during the day and you'll feel better in the long run.

If you've heeded these tips and you still have trouble sleeping or you are excessively tired during the day, it may be time to see a doctor. See Remedy 3 for advice on seeking medical treatment for sleep problems.

2

RECOGNIZE DAYTIME SYMPTOMS.

While symptoms of sleep disturbances often occur at night, the most important clues to sleep-related illness may occur during the day. Fatigue, depression, irritability, and lack of concentration are among the effects of disturbed or poor quality sleep. Because there are many other causes for these complaints, poor sleep is often overlooked as a possible factor.

The most common symptom of poor quality sleep is sleepiness during the day. In its most severe form, this sleepiness can cause you to doze at the wheel, at work, or in other inappropriate places. Sleepiness is still significant but is less serious when you fall asleep at movies, the theatre, or concerts. You may also experience milder sleepiness—where you feel drowsy but do not actually drift off into sleep.

People whose abnormal sleepiness interferes with their daytime routine or causes near-accidents should consult a doctor. They may have a sleep disorder, such as *sleep apnea* or *narcolepsy*. In sleep apnea, pauses in breathing lasting up to one minute or more can occur. These pauses may happen several times in a single night. Each time a breathing pause occurs, the sleeper is briefly awakened, making sleep extremely fragmented.

Another well-known sleep disorder is narcolepsy. A person with narcolepsy experiences uncontrollable sleepiness during the day. The individual may sleep awhile and awake feeling refreshed, but sleepiness returns an hour or two later.

Sleep disorders such as narcolepsy and sleep apnea can improve with treatment. Unfortunately, many people with mild to moderate sleepiness do not seek medical help. But with a proper evaluation by a physician, these drowsy people could, in most cases, find their sleepiness greatly reduced or even eliminated.

It's easy to understand why a person might not make the connection between daytime sleepiness and poor sleep. The sleeper may be totally unaware his or her sleep is poor. Sleep apnea, for example, can cause several *hundred* brief awakenings in a single night—yet the individual believes he or she sleeps soundly. Even those of us without sleep problems experience many such awakenings during the night. Like persons with sleep apnea, we don't remember the awakenings because they are so brief and nothing significant takes place when they occur to make us remember.

Some people truly do sleep well at night but still report daytime sleepiness. In these people, the sleep-producing part of the brain overpowers the part of the brain that keeps them awake. Sleep specialists treat these conditions even though sleep at night is not usually affected.

Is the sleepiness you experience during the day abnormal? If you are falling asleep while driving or when at work, seek medical advice immediately. A little drowsiness in the afternoon is normal; more than that suggests a sleep disorder. Mild to moderate sleepiness or symptoms of depression, irritability, or low energy could also signify something is wrong with your sleep. Remember, there is nothing normal about falling asleep when you wish to stay awake. And older people should understand that increased daytime sleepiness is not simply a normal part of the aging process.

Excessive daytime sleepiness can and should be treated, and the time to get treatment is before it becomes a major problem.

3

SEE A DOCTOR.

So you're having a problem with sleep. But when is the time to see the doctor, and which doctor should you see?

You should seek medical help when your sleep problem persists about three weeks. Of course, if the problem is severe, it may be reasonable to consult a physician sooner. For example, someone who gets fewer than three hours of sleep each night definitely should not wait three weeks before discussing the problem with a doctor.

Problems with daytime sleepiness also demand attention. The most common cause of daytime sleepiness is not getting enough sleep at night. In this case, the first step is not a trip to the doctor but an attempt to increase the amount of sleep you get at night. But if you are falling asleep or drifting off at inappropriate times (at work or when driving), then it is wise to seek medical attention. Such major daytime sleepiness is a serious symptom that should never be ignored.

Snoring and other breathing irregularities in sleep are also signs that point straight to the doctor's office. Snoring can be a social problem, a medical problem, or both. Loud, uneven snoring is the main complaint in sleep apnea, a potentially dangerous condition in which breathing can actually stop for one minute or more during sleep. Sleep-related breathing problems, such as sleep apnea and snoring, almost always improve with treatment, so a visit to the doctor is usually a step toward a rapid cure.

For sleepwalking, another common sleep disorder, age is the most important factor to consider before seeking medical care. Sleepwalking in children is very common, and medical treatment is not necessary unless the behavior is particularly frequent, disruptive, or potentially dangerous. But adults do not normally walk in their sleep. A consultation with a doctor is probably advisable for anyone older than 14 years of age who still walks in his or her sleep. Also seek a physician's advice when sleepwalking occurs for the first time in an adult. In this age group, sleepwalking could be the sign of a more serious medical condition.

If you decide to see a doctor, who should it be? Usually, it's reasonable to start with your family doctor. He or she will take a history of your sleep problem, conduct a physical examination, and order routine blood tests to rule out most medical problems. Should the results of these tests be negative, a referral to a sleep specialist may be the next step.

You should consider several factors when looking for a sleep specialist. First, make sure he or she has the proper credentials. Sleep specialists should be board certified in sleep medicine. Sleep doctors often have training in a second area: psychiatry, neurology, or internal medicine.

If your doctor refers you to a sleep center for diagnosis, the center should be accredited by the American Sleep Disorders Association (ASDA). The ASDA is the professional organization for sleep medicine in the United States. Each accredited laboratory is inspected every five years to ensure it meets certain standards set by the ASDA. Sleep centers that are not accredited may or may not adhere to guidelines established by the ASDA. Be wary if you receive a recommendation for sleep studies performed in your home. These tests have serious limitations and are frequently performed by those with inadequate training.

RECOGNIZE THE CONNECTION BETWEEN MOOD AND SLEEP.

Mood and sleep are often closely related. Poor sleep can cause depression, anxiety, irritability, and even changes in personality, and depression, anxiety, and other psychological problems can cause poor sleep. Sometimes both of these processes can occur at once, producing a snowball effect: Depression can cause poor sleep which then makes the depression worse. Or, disturbed sleep can lead to anxiety, which disturbs sleep even more. Understanding the possible connection between sleep disorders and mood disorders can help you get to the root of both problems.

Do you lack energy and self-esteem, have feelings of sadness and hopelessness, and find yourself withdrawing from friends and family? You may be experiencing depression. Problems getting to sleep, sleeping too long, and waking frequently during the night, especially between 3:00 and 5:00 A.M., are also symptoms of depression. Symptoms of anxiety include a racing heart, sweating palms, shortness of breath, muscle tension, and irritability. If you're anxious, you may find you can't still your thoughts or relax enough to sleep restfully.

Stress may also impact sleep. Insomnia is a common response to stress and, if not too severe, is actually considered normal. Remember that happy occasions, including weddings, vacations, and parties, often involve a certain amount of anxiety or stress that may affect sleep quality. Insomnia related to these kinds of events usually goes away when the event is over.

If you have trouble sleeping consider the possibility that a mood disorder may play a role. One type of mood disorder, manic-depressive disorder, can produce an extreme form of insomnia in which the individual sleeps only four hours each night—or even less. The sleeplessness causes an exaggerated and potentially harmful sense of euphoria rather than sadness.

Some people use sleep as an escape from emotional distress and spend a large portion of the day in bed. Under these circumstances, sleep can occupy 12 hours of the day or more. Psychiatrists call this type of sleep pattern atypical depression. Such a pattern shows just how closely mood can be tied to sleep.

Sleep disorders can also lead to mood disorders. If you've been told you're a snorer, you might also experience sleep apnea, a condition in which breathing actually stops in sleep. Sleep apnea can cause many different daytime symptoms, including depression. Restlessness or leg jerks in sleep could be a sign of restless legs syndrome or periodic movements in sleep (see Remedy 10). Both these conditions can dramatically alter the way you feel during the day.

If sleep problems persist, you should make an appointment with your doctor to determine if a medical problem is involved (see Remedy 3 for advice on when to seek help). If your doctor gives you a clean bill of health, consider consulting a counselor or therapist for help coping with a possible mood disorder. Ask your doctor for a referral to a qualified therapist. Also talk to friends who have received counseling for their recommendations on therapists.

5

SNORE NO MORE.

It has been said, "Laugh and the world laughs with you, snore and you sleep alone." But snoring is no laughing matter when your bed partner sounds like a chain saw at night and you can't get any sleep. The problem can severely strain relationships and force couples to sleep in separate rooms. Very loud snoring has actually been used as grounds for divorce in some states.

Hundreds of patents have been filed with the United States patent office for devices that supposedly cure snoring. Until recently, most were failures. But now a variety of effective techniques, appliances, and procedures are available to eliminate or greatly reduce snoring. Some are simple techniques you can try on your own.

- Avoid alcohol at night. Alcohol relaxes the throat muscles, increasing the snoring. If you stop drinking a few hours before bed, your bed partner may notice a big difference.

- Lose weight—even as little as five or ten pounds. Many people notice the snoring gets better or worse as they lose or gain weight. Unfortunately, weight loss does not reduce snoring in everyone. Also, losing weight (and keeping it off) is more easily said than done.

- Change sleeping position. You may have noticed your bed partner snores more often or more heavily when he sleeps on his back. Some couples resort to the "elbow technique," that is, one bed partner elbows the other onto his or her side when the snoring begins. Happily, there is a less painful method available when the snoring is position-related. If you affix a bulky object to the back of a nightshirt or pajama top, you can restrict sleeping position to the side or stomach. Antisnoring shirts that use this principle are now available. You can make a homemade version by sewing a sock onto the back of a T-shirt and placing a few tennis balls, large pieces of styrofoam, or other light, bulky material in the sock. This "ball-on-back" shirt prevents most people from sleeping on their back and can lead to a snoreless night.

Other methods to reduce snoring require a doctor's care. In recent years, surgeons have developed surgical procedures performed on the upper airway to treat snoring. The standard procedure is UPPP, (uvulopalatopharyngoplasty). UPPP is to the upper airway what a face-lift is to an aging face. Fleshy folds of extra tissue in the throat are removed, which opens up the breathing passages. When air moves over these folds as you breathe, they vibrate, causing the clatter we call snoring. Removing these tissues often puts an end to snoring.

Laser surgery is the newest approach to the treatment of snoring. Unlike conventional surgery, laser surgery does not require a hospital admission or the use of general anaesthesia. It does require several office visits, usually spaced about one month apart. After each treatment, the patient goes home, typically with no discomfort other than a sore throat. Because laser surgery is very new, doctors do not have definite success rates. Nevertheless, early results are promising, and more and more surgeons are performing the operation. Surgery on the nasal passages also sometimes lessens snoring. An ear, nose, and throat doctor or sleep specialist can advise which procedure is best for you.

Because snoring is produced in the upper airway, changing the position of the jaw, tongue, and other oral structures can change the sounds produced by breathing in sleep. A device called a mandibular advancement oral appliance produces just such shifts in position. The appliance looks like a protective mouthpiece worn by a boxer or football player but is custom-molded to fit the individual's teeth. It works by pulling the lower jaw forward and opening up the breathing passages. Most snorers who use an appliance report they are silent or at least much more quiet when they sleep.

Another type of oral appliance holds the tongue forward, preventing it from blocking the airway. This tongue-retaining device may be less comfortable than the mandibular advancement appliance but in some cases is more effective. Your doctor can help you decide which appliance will offer the best results.

Finally, a note to those of you kept awake by the snores of your loved ones: Listen for irregularities in the snoring. Loud snorts, pauses in breathing, and gasps may indicate sleep apnea, a potentially serious medical problem that requires a visit to the doctor.

SEE M.D. FOR TOO MANY NIGHTTIME BATHROOM TRIPS.

Nothing will force you out of your nice warm bed into that icebox you call your bedroom. But then you sense that unmistakable pressure, and you stumble from your warm bed across the cold floor to the bathroom.

While many people sleep through the night without interruption, many others must get up one or more times to urinate. Trips to the bathroom at night may simply mean you consumed too much liquid in the evening. And, certainly, the need to urinate once during a night's sleep is normal and not cause for concern. But if you must get up two or more times every night, there may be a problem.

First, getting up disturbs your sleep. (But fighting the urge to get up isn't a good solution: The discomfort of pressure on the bladder makes sleep light and of poor quality.) When several such awakenings occur in a single night, the loss of sleep time adds up. You will surely feel the consequences the next day.

But more important than the loss of sleep, several trips to the bathroom at night could

signal a medical problem. Excessive urina-
tion at night (*nocturia*) is a common symptom
of several conditions, including diabetes.
In men, an enlarged prostate gland (a
problem that occurs in most men as they age)
is very often the problem. An enlarged
prostate can also be a warning sign of
prostate cancer and should be evaluated
promptly. In women, urinary tract infections
frequently cause nocturia.

Drinking alcohol in the evening can be a factor in nocturia. And many prescription drugs
have nocturia as a side effect. Because nocturia has so many causes, a doctor's evaluation
is important. Afterward, your doctor may refer
you to a urologist or other specialist.

If you have to use the bathroom at night,
use only the minimum amount of light to nav-
igate. Too much bright light may make it difficult to return to sleep. If getting up is a
nightly occurrence for you, light the path to
the bathroom with night-lights so you don't
have to turn on any lights.

7

LIFT YOUR HEAD TO EASE HEARTBURN.

Most of us have had the burning or gnawing sensation in the middle of the chest that signifies a case of heartburn. Despite its name, heartburn has nothing to do with the heart. It is really caused when the esophagus, the tube that connects the mouth to the stomach, is exposed to the highly acidic contents of the stomach. When this occurs, the material in the stomach is said to "reflux" into the esophagus.

You may not even realize the reflux is occurring because it can occur without the telltale "burn." Other common signs of reflux include the following:

- A taste of bile. When the contents of the small intestine move backward all the way into the mouth, you may awake with a bitter or sour taste in your mouth.

- Coughing that wakes you up. Should the acid contents of your stomach reflux into the breathing passages, the vocal cords can go into spasm and cause blockage of the airway. This causes intense coughing fits.

Reflux is most apt to occur when you are lying down. In this position, the force of gravity does not help move food from the stomach into the small intestine, where it is supposed to go. Because we generally sleep in a horizontal position, reflux is most common at night.

There are many causes of reflux, but all involve the backward movement of partially digested food from the stomach. The contents of the stomach, which are highly acidic, leak past the valve that separates the stomach from the esophagus. While the stomach has a special lining that protects it from the strong acid, the esophagus does not; thus you feel the acid's effects as a burning sensation in your chest.

You should consult your doctor if you regularly experience reflux. Your doctor may recommend you make some of the following changes in your diet and your lifestyle.

- Avoid alcohol.

- Avoid heavily spiced foods and other common heartburn-causing foods such as chocolate, peppermint, and coffee.

- Control your weight.

- Manage stress.

- Do not eat heavy meals within three hours of going to bed.

- Do not lie down after eating.

Another simple and safe remedy to curb reflux is to raise the head of your bed. Tilting the bed allows gravity to help the stomach contents follow their natural path into the small intestine.

You can use several methods to elevate your bed. When possible, consider using an electrically adjustable bed. Although these beds can be expensive, some insurance plans cover them if a medical condition requires their use.

An alternative is to place blocks underneath the legs of the headboard. Begin with just a small amount of lift; a few inches may be sufficient. If you use supporting blocks, be sure they are wide enough to provide a safe and secure base. If the bed is on wheels, make sure it cannot roll off the blocks.

Using several pillows to elevate your head may seem like a good (and simpler) idea. But it's too easy to roll off the pillows during sleep, thus defeating the purpose. A more certain technique such as the electric bed or tilting the entire bed is required.

8

DON'T RELY ON OVER-THE-COUNTER CURES.

Almost everyone at one time or another has difficulty falling asleep or staying asleep. When the problem persists for more than one or two days, you may consider taking a sleeping pill. Since prescription drugs are expensive and usually involve a visit to the doctor, you may decide an easier solution is to choose one of the numerous over-the-counter sleeping aids.

Over-the-counter sleeping pills, or hypnotics, as they're sometimes called, can be very useful for the treatment of occasional sleeplessness. Take care when using them, because most of these sleeping pills contain an antihistamine. Many antihistamines produce drowsiness and so are used as a remedy for insomnia. While they're generally safe, adverse reactions to these drugs do occur. Don't think that just because you can get these pills without a prescription they are completely without side effects.

The ideal use of these pills is for insomnia that occurs sporadically and for short periods. For example, should you have trouble sleeping the night before the league bowling championship, consider a sleeping pill. But consult your doctor if sleep problems persist; those that last for weeks or months require a doctor's treatment. (See Remedy 3 for more information on when to see a doctor.)

Do not take over-the-counter sleeping aids during the day. All over-the-counter hypnotics produce decreased mental alertness. If you have an occupation that requires you to be on call, you should consider the potential hazards if you're called to work after taking a sleep aid. Do not use these drugs unless absolutely necessary.

Some people still experience sleepiness more than 24 hours after taking the pills. Be sure to consider this possibility, especially when you use an over-the-counter hypnotic for the first time.

If you use one of these agents and it does not help you sleep, stop taking it. Many people continue taking these pills even though they clearly don't work.

If you use over-the-counter sleeping pills properly, they can be very helpful for occasional bouts of poor sleep. Remember to always read label directions before taking these or any over-the-counter medications.

WEAN SLOWLY FROM SLEEPING PILLS.

As a rule, do not stop taking prescription sleeping pills suddenly. You could experience a worsening of the sleep problem, or *rebound insomnia*. Rebound insomnia occurs because your body is accustomed to the pill and depends on it for sleep. If you take these pills every night, they may also have a calming effect during the day (most prescription sleeping pills are actually mild tranquilizers). When you stop, they can cause *rebound anxiety* when you are awake.

You can reduce the effects of rebound insomnia and anxiety by gradually cutting back your use of the sleeping pills. If you take less and less over a period of time, your body can adjust to their absence. Talk with your doctor about a schedule for reducing the dosage. If you follow your doctor's instructions, you can stop taking the sleeping pills with a minimum of effort or discomfort. This advice does not apply to most nonprescription sleeping pills, which are not addictive and do not have rebound effects. See Remedy 8 for advice on over-the-counter sleep agents.

CALM RESTLESS LEGS.

For most of us, the evening is a time for rest and relaxation. For others, however, this is a time of special anxiety. As the evening hours progress, these people feel more and more restless. They fidget, bounce their legs, rub their calves, walk around. By bedtime the sensation is maddening; the urge to move their legs, overwhelming. Sleep is the farthest thought from their minds. All they can think about is the weird feeling in their legs.

These individuals have *restless legs syndrome,* a medical condition that can cause severe discomfort and insomnia. The main symptom is a deep, restless feeling in the calves and thighs. (One patient said it feels as though worms are crawling around in her legs.) Though it is worse at night, the restlessness may even occur during the day.

Restless legs are often accompanied by *periodic movements* in sleep. Periodic movements are leg jerks that occur at 60- to 90-second intervals, often causing hundreds of brief arousals from sleep. Although the sleeper doesn't remember these arousals, their effect is often daytime sleepiness.

Consult your doctor if you suspect you have restless legs or periodic movements. Both conditions can be treated with medication. But medication can only help prevent restless legs syndrome; it cannot eliminate it. Unfortunately, no other treatment methods have proven helpful in all persons with the condition. What may provide relief for some may not have any effect for others. For example, some people with restless legs claim the condition worsens after a day of strenuous activity; others say exercise early in the day helps. If you find a remedy that works for you, by all means, use it.

Aspirin, acetaminophen, or ibuprofen can help relieve some of the discomfort. Over-the-counter or prescription sleeping pills are not a solution, however. Some people find heat applications or a warm bath helps. Massage may also help a little. Some people place a pillow between their knees to be more comfortable when they sleep. You can also try reducing or eliminating caffeine intake to see if the condition improves. Do not use alcohol to try to calm your restless legs; it will only disturb your sleep more.

DON'T IGNORE SLEEPWALKING.

Sleepwalking is one of the most mysterious of the sleep disorders. Until recently, doctors had little understanding of these strange episodes, and there was not much in the way of treatment. But new research is beginning to unlock the secrets of sleepwalking, and almost all cases can be successfully treated.

We now know there are two main types of sleepwalking. The first type, which primarily affects children, takes place during the deepest part of nondreaming, or *non-REM,* sleep. REM stands for the *rapid eye movement* that occurs in dreaming sleep. Non-REM sleepwalking occurs when the brain is half awake and half asleep. It happens most often in children because their sleep is much deeper than the average adult's (see Remedy 49 for how to handle sleepwalking in children). Almost all children experience this type of sleepwalking, and most outgrow the problem by adolescence.

The second type of sleepwalking occurs during the dreaming, or REM, phase of sleep. Called *REM behavior disorder,* sleepwalking of this type is actually an attempt by sleepers to act out their dreams. REM behavior disorder usually occurs in middle age or later. Because people with this condition often move about vigorously or may even become violent in response to threatened harm in their dreams, bed partners often suffer the brunt of this condition and are kicked, punched, or slapped.

Follow this advice for sleepwalking:

- If you are an adult who is experiencing sleepwalking episodes and you have previously walked during sleep, consider seeing your doctor to determine if treatment is necessary.

- If you are an adult who never before walked during sleep but you have recently started, you should definitely seek a doctor's advice. While the sudden onset of sleepwalking in an adult is usually just a variant of non-REM sleepwalking or REM behavior disorder, occasionally a more serious medical problem is the cause.

- When sleepwalking is frequent, the sleepwalker's behavior is vigorous or violent, or injury occurs to you or a bed partner as a result of sleepwalking, you should consult a doctor without delay.

Medication to treat both non-REM sleepwalking and REM behavior disorder is available. These drugs are generally effective in ensuring that sleep is safe, sound, and confined to the bedroom. Your doctor can advise you about the best approach to managing out-of-bed experiences. While psychological intervention, such as therapy, is usually not necessary for such events, do not dismiss the possible role of stress. If stress appears to be a significant factor in adult sleepwalking, seek advice from your physician or a therapist.

Regardless of whether you receive treatment, you should take precautions against potential accident or injury. For example, lock bedroom windows, remove sharp objects from the bedside, and restrict access to stairs or other hazards.

A note to housemates of sleepwalkers: If a sleepwalker is very active, try to keep obstacles out of his or her path. In some cases, you may be able to lead the sleepwalker back to bed. If, however, a sleepwalker is violent, stay out of the way. Do not risk injury attempting to wake the sleeper. Do seek medical treatment for the sleepwalker as soon as possible.

RELAX BEFORE BED.

To people who fall asleep quickly and sleep soundly through the night, the idea of needing to prepare for sleep may seem odd. But, in fact, to fall asleep quickly and stay asleep during the night, your body needs to be primed for that period of inactivity.

Preparation for sleep can actually take place over the entire day. Many of the techniques in this book relate to ways in which daytime activities can be modified to improve sleep. But the hour before bedtime is the most critical. Used properly, the time right before bedtime can serve as a buffer between the stressful, anxiety-provoking events of the day and a restful sleep at night. But if it is not used properly, that last hour can set the stage for a long night of tossing and turning.

The key to preparing for sleep is to establish an atmosphere of peace and calm. The first step is to try to forget the problems of the day. If this seems impossible, bear in mind you won't solve them in that hour before sleep anyway. Ease your mind and body with quiet yet pleasurable activities. You will create a sense of inner well-being that allows sleep to come quickly and easily. The following are a few suggestions to help you prepare yourself for sleep:

- If the weather and noise level in your neighborhood permit, sit quietly outside on the porch or balcony. Try to keep your mind away from the trials and tribulations of the day.

- Read to relax, but you should select your reading material with care. A treatise on the microeconomics of sixteenth century Europe would be a fine choice, while a horror novel or thrilling murder mystery might not exactly prove soothing. Remember the key: Good, but dull.

- Watch television if it helps you relax. But, again, its effect depends upon the programming you select. As a general rule of thumb, steer clear of action-adventure programs; choose news and talk shows. And make sure the television is in a room other than the bedroom.

- Listen to music. Choose the type of music that relaxes you. Some people find more relaxation in the Rolling Stones than in Mozart. If you fit this category, listening to rock music will help your sleep more than a flock of classical flutists.

- Try meditation or prayer. These activities, which help many people relax, can also help you come to peace with whatever is on your mind.

- Relaxing your mind is obviously important, but don't neglect your body. Try a warm bath or—even better—a massage. But not all massage is equal in sleep preparation. Shiatsu style massage, which involves vigorous manipulation of the muscles, can relieve tension but may be too stimulating for some people. A better bet might be Swedish massage, which uses long, smooth strokes to gently knead the muscles. Any massage should concentrate on the neck and back; those areas are most affected by stress.

If you set aside the hour before bedtime to relax—whatever method of relaxation you use—your sleep will be enhanced. It may take some discipline to set aside your problems and limit yourself to quiet activities, but the end result is worth the effort.

13

ESTABLISH PRESLEEP RITUALS.

Another way to help prepare yourself for sleep is to adopt presleep rituals—rituals that signal your body and mind that it's time to sleep.

You probably already have some of these rituals, even if you haven't realized it. Brushing and flossing your teeth, lowering the thermostat, and setting your alarm clock are all part of your evening routine. To help you get to sleep, you should perform these activities in the same manner and order every night.

Before you get into bed, turn off the lights in your house, turn on any night-lights, check the locks and the stove, and close the windows. Performing these rituals helps create a sense of security—if you don't feel secure, you'll find it difficult to relax. Establishing presleep rituals such as these also provides closure to your day and effectively sends the message to your mind and body that it's bed—and sleep—time.

14

DON'T GO TO BED ANGRY!

You've just gotten into a political argument. You race home mumbling curses to yourself. Flying into your bedroom like a whirlwind, you try to get ready for bed. You're glowing with anger. You lie down on the bed and repeatedly slam your fist into your pillow as you try to find a comfortable position. But you can't fall asleep . . . you're on fire.

Too often people go to bed when their mind is a raging fury, agonizing over events of the day. Don't make this mistake. You don't want your bed to be a place for anger, worry, and problems. Your bedroom should produce a feeling of peace and contentment.

When your emotions have boiled over make an effort to calm yourself before you try to go to sleep.

Take the time before bed to relax both your mind and body. Use one or two of the techniques described in Remedy 12, even if you're going to bed late. The hour or so you spend to relax could save you hours of sleeplessness at night and sleepiness during the day.

15

DON'T WORRY ABOUT SLEEP.

If you have insomnia, you may spend your day worrying about how you're going to get a good night's sleep. Anxiety builds through the afternoon and evening, and it's no wonder that by bedtime you're a nervous wreck. Simply put, worrying about sleep is rarely productive. It only results in more stress, more anxiety, and more insomnia.

As you lie in bed and try to sleep, keep your thoughts pleasant and relaxed. If you're having trouble keeping your thoughts on pleasant subjects, see Remedy 12 for suggestions to still your mind and your body.

Remember, almost everyone has some nights when sleep is light, fragmented, or just plain difficult to get. For most people, the normal sleep pattern returns after a few days. But excessive concern about your sleep can actually cause enough stress to lead to prolonged insomnia!

So save your worries for other matters. Worrying can't solve a sleep problem, but it could make it much worse.

DON'T TRY TOO HARD.

While lying in bed, tossing and turning, we may concentrate on trying to sleep, perhaps even repeating over and over, "I will go to sleep, I will go to sleep." Our hope is that by sheer force of effort, we can put our mind and body to rest and fall asleep.

But sleep is unlike most activities in life. While trying harder is often the surest path to success in business, sports, or other waking activities, it is the surest path to failure in getting to sleep. Attempting to force yourself to sleep simply won't work. It only increases energy and anxiety levels. Sleep is most easily achieved in an atmosphere of total relaxation. Your mind should be empty of thought or turned to soothing and calming thoughts. Your body should be relaxed, your muscles free of tension. (Follow the techniques suggested in Remedy 12 to relax.) Thinking about sleep only guarantees a long, restless night.

Sleep can be a welcome release from your cares if you allow it to be. Remember, a good night's sleep is your best weapon to fight the battles of the coming day.

AVOID PROCRASTINATION.

Many of us live by the motto "Why do today what I can put off until tomorrow?" But putting work or projects off almost always has bad consequences, one of which is disturbed sleep. Falling asleep is difficult when thoughts of unfinished business drift in and out of your mind. Tasks left undone can even intrude into your dreams at night and, in extreme cases, lead to nightmares.

Avoiding procrastination takes some discipline. Sometimes making a "to do" list for the day helps. But attend to the most difficult and unpleasant tasks first. Leaving unpleasant chores for later in the day is the first step in not doing them at all. And even the best of intentions can be waylaid by unexpected events.

Always try to finish what you start. An incomplete job will occupy your mind and make relaxing difficult.

It's also useful to make schedules and stick to them. When promised work is late, it only becomes more difficult to face.

If you apply a little self-discipline, you may find it easier to relax at night.

DON'T OBSESS OVER DREAMS.

Dreams are a controversial subject even among most sleep researchers. The father of psychoanalysis, Sigmund Freud, believed dreams to be of crucial importance to psychological well-being. He called them "the royal road to the unconscious," meaning they are the key to unlocking our innermost thoughts and feelings. On the other hand, some scientists today attach almost no importance to dreams. They claim dreams are only random thoughts drifting into our minds during sleep; they have no serious relationship to our waking life, and dream analysis has no value whatsoever.

The truth probably lies somewhere between these two extremes. Almost all dreams tell us something about ourselves, and some may have great significance. Nearly everyone, though, has had simple, unemotional dreams about routine matters in everyday life. It may or may not be useful to look for hidden meanings in dreams of winning the lottery or pitching a no-hitter in the World Series.

Virtually everyone dreams every night. Drug use, prior sleep patterns, illness, and other factors may alter the length, frequency, and time of occurrence of dreams, but a truly dreamless sleep is unusual. Most people will have four or five dream, or REM (rapid eye movement), periods each night during which one or more dreams will occur. We only remember dreams if we awaken during the dream or very shortly thereafter. Thus, people who sleep soundly through REM periods will have little or no dream recall.

Most people find even casual analysis of their dreams helpful in understanding themselves and solving problems of everyday life. Bits and pieces of information come together in unexpected ways during dreaming, often leading to waking insights.

Dreams can be divided into four categories. *Lucid dreams* are those in which the dreamer can control the action as if he or she were awake. The dreamer can make characters in the dream appear and disappear or shift the action to any place or time. All elements of the dream are under the dreamer's complete control.

Recurrent dreams are another interesting phenomenon. Usually these dreams reveal psychological issues and can be interesting for an individual to ponder. Some repeating dreams may have roots in basic human biology; for example, when we enter the state of sleep in which we dream, our muscles become paralyzed. The paralysis is very real—it protects us from acting out dreams when we sleep. Even though we are asleep, we may have some awareness of this paralysis, which may cause our minds to create dreams in which we are trapped and unable to escape—one of the most common themes in recurrent dreams.

Even *nightmares* can be useful and revealing. A nightmare is a very frightening or disquieting dream. It, too, can reveal conflicts, problems, and issues the dreamer might not have been aware of otherwise. Once you recover from the acute anxiety a nightmare creates, try to store it away until morning and go back to sleep. In the morning, give some thought to the dream's meaning; try to benefit from this movie shown to you. Treat recurrent dreams the same way.

When children have nightmares, they usually just require a parent's comfort. Nightmares get less and less frequent as children get older and should occur only very occasionally by adolescence. Frequent nightmares in any age group may suggest overwhelming stress or problems that require medical intervention. Consult with your doctor or a sleep center for guidance.

Stress is not the only cause of bad dreams. Medical conditions and medications can contribute. Antidepressants, for example, commonly cause bad dreams, but you should consider any medication you've recently begun taking as the possible cause. Frequent bad dreams, no matter what the cause, are very distressing. They disturb sleep and may even make you fearful of sleep. Bring the problem to the attention of your doctor.

In children, nightmares should be distinguished from *night terrors*. Night terrors are similar to sleepwalking in that the dreamer is half awake and half asleep. But instead of walking around, the child screams. Usually the child has no recall of the content of the dream, a feature that distinguishes night terrors from nightmares. Children often experience terrors; they usually outgrow them by adolescence. Generally, night terrors do not indicate any psychological problems, but it's a good idea to mention them to your doctor. Occasionally, a combination of terrors and sleepwalking can occur, and the child runs around screaming. This activity can be somewhat dangerous for the child and may require medication management for a short while. When the problem persists into late adolescence or the early 20s, medication can often be very useful and protective for the dreamer and his or her roommates.

We all dream three, four, or five times a night in 5- to 45-minute discrete episodes. When you feel as if you have been dreaming all night, you have just had especially vivid dreams. Such dreams can leave you feeling drained in the morning. Approach these and others dreams the same way. Remember them, consider them, and mine them for useful ideas. If you have some intuition a particular dream is important, give it further thought. Relate the dream content to your current life situation and see if it offers any insight or direction. Use your dreams as one piece of information in the great puzzle of life, but do not rely on them exclusively when making critical decisions. When kept in proper perspective, dreams can be an enjoyable and useful addition to the pleasures of waking life.

19

EXERCISE EARLY.

For many people, a long run, bicycle ride, or workout at the gym follows a long day at work. Because such vigorous exercise leads to physical fatigue, it would seem sleep should follow naturally and easily. True, after an hour of intense, heart-pounding exercise, you will probably feel exhausted. You may want nothing more than to crawl into the bedroom, throw on your pajamas, and pass out on your nice, soft bed. But vigorous exercise right before bedtime does not improve your sleep. Though you may feel tired, your body is actually revved up. Your heart, brain, and other organs, stimulated by the exercise, need time to cool down.

There is a way to get the exercise you need and sleep better: Exercise earlier in the day. Daily exercise helps relieve inner tensions, release energy, and improve sleep. Studies show athletes generally sleep more soundly than nonathletes. But don't get the idea one day of mad exercise will benefit you; it is the fitness that regular exercise produces that helps. Physical exhaustion from overdoing it only makes sleep worse.

Of course, some people simply can't fit morning or afternoon exercise into their schedule. But you can adapt your exercise routine to your schedule. Instead of a late evening jog, consider milder forms of exercise. Try a walk instead (but don't make it too brisk). Other effective exercises use relaxation techniques and, thus, provide a smooth transition from the daytime to the night. Yoga, which involves stretching and meditation, is an example. Tai chi is a martial art that involves a series of movements performed slowly to remove stress. Both yoga and tai chi relax the body but do not require tremendous physical effort.

So do yourself a favor. Schedule 30 to 45 minutes of exercise at least three or four times a week. (Put it on your to-do list; make it a regular part of your routine—just like brushing your teeth.) Walk to work or walk the dog. Jog, jump rope, dance, or swim. Choose whatever activity you enjoy. Just make it a habit. Regular exercise can help you feel better, look better, and sleep better.

20

BE CAREFUL WITH CAFFEINE.

Coffee is such a part of our daily routine that we call our midmorning and midafternoon break periods "coffee breaks." For many, a day without several cups of coffee is nearly unthinkable.

The ingredient in coffee that helps us to wake up and stay alert is caffeine. Though caffeine's effects can be useful, caffeine has the unwanted side effect of disturbing sleep. On average, people who have even two cups of coffee a day spend a longer time trying to get to sleep. They may also awaken more often during the night. Increased heart rate, muscle tension or twitches, headaches, and anxiety may also result from too much caffeine. None of these conditions helps you sleep.

One or two cups of coffee in the morning is fine. More than that suggests you're trying to combat too much sleepiness in the day, or you have a bad caffeine habit. And don't be one of those people who says coffee doesn't disturb your sleep. Coffee does disturb sleep, and if you can sleep despite an evening cup, then you are too tired. Even when you're this tired, coffee lightens sleep, but you may not be aware of it. Overuse of caffeine can start a cycle of poor sleep, tiredness in the day, use of caffeine to combat the tiredness, poor sleep, and so on. What you may not have realized is that because you may develop some tolerance to the alerting effects of caffeine (but not to its sleep-disturbing effects), the less you use regularly, the more it will provide a boost when you really need it.

Caffeine's effect can last much longer than you think, so try not to have any within six hours of your bedtime. Also, don't underestimate the caffeine content of other products. Regular tea and cola contain caffeine, and some over-the-counter medications have large amounts of caffeine that can also reduce the quality of your sleep.

SNACK LIGHTLY BEFORE BEDTIME.

You've just finished a 36 course meal and topped it off with a pint of ice cream. Sure, you *feel* sleepy, but ingesting such a heavy meal actually stimulates your body and may give you a stomachache—both make sleep quite difficult. But then again, you can't go to sleep on an empty stomach. Hunger is a definite cause for insomnia. And if you must get up in the middle of the night to fix yourself a sandwich, you may find getting back to sleep a chore.

The solution is quite simple: Have a light snack about 30 minutes before you retire. Studies show a quick bite to eat before bed can help you sleep more soundly. Preferably, you should have this snack in the kitchen: Crumbs in bed are definitely not a recipe for sound sleep.

What you eat is almost as important as how much and when. Steer clear of foods that contain the flavor enhancer monosodium glutamate (MSG), a substance associated with insomnia. Also make sure to avoid anything that might contain caffeine, such as soda, tea, coffee, and chocolate. Contrary to popular belief, alcohol does not help you sleep (see Remedy 23). And avoid fried and spicy foods that could produce heartburn and keep you awake. What should you eat instead? Whatever works for you.

Try some of the natural sleep-inducers. Some people find L-tryptophan, a naturally occurring substance, helps them sleep more soundly. Milk (warm, if possible), cottage cheese, cashews, chicken, turkey, soybeans, and tuna are especially good food sources of this compound. (Be aware that the Food and Drug Administration has banned tryptophan in pill form because harmful contaminants found in one manufacturer's product caused a serious blood disorder.)

Others find a snack high in carbohydrates and low in protein does the trick. A sandwich or toast, a bowl of cereal, crackers, or other high-carbohydrate foods might be a good choice for you. Some people also swear by herbal teas, such as chamomile, to induce sleepiness.

QUIT SMOKING!

Smoking cigarettes not only causes a countless number of diseases, it keeps you awake. Studies show heavy smokers are at greater risk of insomnia than nonsmokers. It takes them longer to fall asleep, and they experience more awakenings during the night. (We don't usually remember these awakenings, but they do affect how we feel the next day.) Also, if withdrawal symptoms kick in a couple hours after your last cigarette, you might get up at 2:00 A.M. searching for another smoke.

Even light smokers, people who smoke an average of one pack a day, are awake a larger percentage of the night than nonsmokers.

If you decide to quit smoking, you may have some trouble sleeping. A regular sleep schedule, a proper diet, exercise, and stress reduction (see Remedy 12) can help you cope with quitting as well as help you get a good night's sleep. You may also want to speak to your doctor about the use of prescription sleeping pills for a week or two.

DON'T DRINK AND SLEEP.

Alcohol is possibly the drug most commonly used to promote drowsiness and enhance sleep—ahead of even prescription and over-the-counter remedies. And it's true that alcohol may help you fall asleep more quickly. Subjects in the sleep laboratory generally pass from wakefulness to light sleep faster after drinking a moderate amount of alcohol. Unfortunately, the effects of alcohol do not persist beyond the first few hours of the night. Research studies have shown that *withdrawal insomnia* occurs: Sleep is actually worse during the second half of the night after consuming one or more presleep drinks. Thus, alcohol's early beneficial effects on sleep are more than offset by its later, sleep-disrupting effects.

Using alcohol as a sleeping aid can lead to other problems, including alcohol overuse or even alcoholism. The process may begin innocently enough—say, with a glass of wine before retiring. But because the alcohol actually causes awakenings during the night, there is a tendency to drink more to suppress these later awakenings. The increased alcohol consumption further disturbs sleep, and a vicious cycle of worsening sleep and more drinking occurs. Over time, a problem with alcohol may develop.

Drinking can also affect a sleeper's breathing. Alcohol consistently makes snoring louder and may cause short pauses in breathing that awaken the sleeper. In a person with sleep apnea, who already has many such pauses during the night, alcohol causes the pauses to become longer and more frequent, and, therefore, more dangerous. When sleep is disturbed by abnormal breathing patterns, decreased alertness, fatigue, and diminished mental sharpness result the following day.

So don't reach for a drink if you can't sleep. Try some of the relaxation techniques outlined in Remedy 12. If you feel you need more help getting to sleep, talk with your doctor about a prescription sleeping pill or try an over-the-counter sleep agent. Follow the label directions and limit use of over-the-counter products to no more than one or two consecutive nights (see Remedy 8 for more information).

TAKE A MORNING WALK.

You probably didn't need this book to tell you that too much light can cause problems getting to sleep and staying asleep. What you may not have known is that exposure to light at other times, particularly in the early morning, can actually help sleep at night.

How does morning light improve sleep? The light resets your biological clocks. These internal clocks are actually areas of the brain that keep time not all that much differently from your wristwatch. Under normal conditions, these biological clocks have a cycle of slightly greater than 24 hours, much like a watch that is running a little too slowly.

Each day the clock must be reset so it runs together with the earth's 24-hour daily rhythm. Research has shown that people who are deprived of light for long periods of time (and thus do not have their biological clocks reset) experience dramatic changes in their sleep, temperature, and hormone cycles.

Although you probably won't be deprived of light for an extended length of time, if your internal clocks are not reset, you may have a tough time falling asleep when you want at night and getting up when you want in the morning.

Many factors can affect our biological clocks, but light is the most important. Timing of the light is crucial; the body clocks are responsive only to sunlight in the early morning between 6:00 and 8:30 A.M. Sunlight later in the day does not provide the same benefit. The type of light also matters, as does the length of exposure. Direct sunlight outdoors for at least one-half hour produces the most benefit. The indoor lighting in a typical home or office has little effect. Specially designed light boxes and visors that simulate light from the sun are now available. They are not used routinely but are sometimes prescribed to treat seasonal affective disorder, or SAD, a form of depression that seems to be triggered by lack of sunlight. SAD gets its name because the depression occurs seasonally—it is linked with the darker winter months.

The effects of sunlight are greatest when combined with physical activity. So take an early morning walk, run, or bicycle ride to help regulate your body's rhythms and help you sleep at night.

BEWARE OF FREELANCE WRITER'S SYNDROME.

Work schedules may vary from person to person, but whether they punch a time clock or have flexible hours, most people have jobs that require their presence at specified times of the day or night. Because our daily activities are generally planned around our work schedules, everything, including sleep, is subject to this routine.

For students, freelance writers, artists, and others, life is very different. Although these people have deadlines, for the most part, they can do their work day or night. But they don't necessarily have work schedules that force any particular bedtime or waking time. For these people, work, sleep, and other activities may occur at any time at all.

While most of us may envy such a lifestyle, it has some definite pitfalls. Our bodies are designed to go to bed and get up at the same time each day. When we have a consistent schedule for sleeping and waking, we sleep more soundly and we are more alert during the daylight hours. A regular schedule helps ensure that our biological clocks, the time-

keepers that are part of our brains, run together with the day-night cycle set by the
earth rotating on its axis. When we sleep at
night one day, during the day the next, and
take several long naps on still another day, our
body clocks shift from their normal rhythms.

While some people can manage with this
type of sleep pattern, most suffer at least some
consequences. They include daytime sleepiness,
insomnia, and increased frequency of stomach
upset, headaches, and other mild illnesses.
Because this syndrome is especially common
among professional writers, it has been given
the name freelance writer's syndrome.

When forced to alter their sleep pattern to
meet outside demands, people on these constantly changing schedules are often unable
to do so. The biggest problem occurs when
they must shift permanently to more conventional sleep hours. Recent college graduates
often encounter this problem when they start
their first full-time job.

The problems associated with this condition provide a valuable lesson: Keep a regular
sleep period. Even if you don't have consistent
work hours, you need to make your sleep-
wake schedule consistent. The following are a
few helpful hints.

- Start by organizing your daytime activities. Set aside certain hours for work and certain hours for recreation, and abide by your schedule.

- If you are a student, try to arrange your schedule so your classes are at the same time each day. A schedule with early morning classes on Monday and Wednesday, afternoon classes on Thursday and Friday, and an evening class on Tuesday almost guarantees your sleep rhythm will be disturbed.

- If you're a freelance professional, assign yourself specific work hours in your home office. Decide what time of day you will work and stick to this schedule. (Let family and friends know what your hours are so you aren't interrupted during this time.) Even if you have to put in long hours on a project with a tight deadline, keep your sleep period as close to your scheduled time as you can.

Not only will a stable rhythm of sleeping and waking improve the quality of your sleep, but it will probably also improve the quality of your work.

SHIFT YOUR HABITS WITH YOUR WORK.

Shift work does not come naturally to us. Our bodies are designed to work in the daylight and on a consistent schedule. Working on artificial schedules with nighttime hours has consequences. People tend to sleep poorly and have decreased alertness in the day. They also have more accidents, work less efficiently, and have increased stress at home.

Rotating shift workers face the biggest problems. Fortunately, there are two rules to make rotating shift work easier:

1. Change from one shift to another as infrequently as possible. Every time you change shifts, your body has to adjust. This adjustment usually causes insomnia and daytime sleepiness and can lead to other illnesses. Obviously, the less often this happens the better.

2. When you must change shifts, the change should occur in this order: day shift to swing shift to night shift. This order follows your body clock's natural tendency to move forward. If you shift in the other di-

rection (day shift to night shift to swing shift), you will find it much harder to adapt to each shift rotation.

If your company does not follow these rules, discuss possible changes with coworkers, union leaders, or supervisors. If you are a manager at a facility that rotates shifts, consider implementing these changes or switching to a system that does not use rotating shifts. Experts who study biological clocks now act as corporate consultants to help companies improve work schedules. Studies show modified schedules that follow these two simple rules can result in improved worker morale, higher productivity, and greater job safety.

Workers on permanent swing shift or the night shift can also face difficulties. If you are a swing shift worker and your shift ends around midnight, try to get to bed by 2:00 A.M. If you sleep until 10:00 A.M., your sleep time will be very close to that of most day shift workers.

The night shift poses a more serious dilemma because a near-normal sleep-wake schedule is virtually impossible. People on the night shift have two choices: sleep right after work or immediately before work. Sleeping during the morning and afternoon makes it difficult to tend to routine business such as banking and shopping. Also, at these times daylight is brightest and street noise is loudest. You may not be able to consistently obtain restful, uninterrupted sleep.

Sleeping in the evening may make it easier to accomplish some routine chores but could prove a hardship in other ways. Because most of the world operates on a 9:00 A.M. to 5:00 P.M. schedule, social activity usually occurs in the evening. This includes time spent with family and friends. If you sleep in the late afternoon and evening, you may have scant opportunity for meals, recreation, or even a quiet evening in front of the television with your loved ones.

Unfortunately, there is no perfect solution for people who regularly work the night shift. Nevertheless, the following guidelines can help:

- Choose a time for sleep that minimizes the separation between you and your family. And set aside some time each day to spend with your children.

- Once you decide when you will sleep, keep that time as consistent as possible—even on weekends or other days off.

- Plan errands ahead, so they don't interfere with sleep. For example, if you sleep right after work, use a bank that has evening hours.

• As a rule, limit sleep to one long block, rather than getting a shorter block with later naps.

By maintaining a regular schedule, you can mitigate the toll of working the night shift.

DON'T DEPRIVE YOURSELF OF SLEEP.

Sleep deprivation is the most common sleep disorder. Virtually everyone goes at least an occasional night without the amount of sleep they need, and many people seem to never get enough. We are all familiar with the symptoms: fatigue, irritability, poor concentration. When we don't get enough sleep, even routine tasks become difficult chores. Simple problems in addition and subtraction suddenly take minutes to solve instead of seconds. As our reflexes slow and attention wavers, a short drive across town becomes as treacherous as walking through a mine field. The sounds of children playing are no longer joyful and welcome, but grate like fingernails scraped across a chalkboard. Perhaps this famous quote says it best: "Fatigue makes cowards of us all."

Unfortunately, the effects of sleep deprivation are not always easy to detect. Poor decision-making, mistakes, and low work efficiency that is actually due to sleep deprivation might be attributed to lack of ability or motivation. But in some jobs the results are clear and sometimes frightening. The *Challenger* space shuttle disaster, in which seven astronauts were killed, was due in part to sleep loss by the project managers. Other industrial accidents, including those at the nuclear reactors at Three Mile Island and Chernobyl, have involved sleep loss. Numerous fatal truck accidents occur each year due to drivers falling asleep at the wheel.

Many people claim they don't have time to sleep as much as they would like. They fail to consider that they work less efficiently and make more mistakes when they have not gotten enough sleep. An extra hour of sleep at night might make the waking day shorter, but the ability to think and act faster will usually more than compensate.

The key is to find out how much sleep your body requires and get that amount every single night. If you get only six hours each night but feel well rested, alert, and awake during the day, then six hours of sleep is all you need. On the other hand, if you're still tired after eight hours of sleep but feel well rested with nine hours, then your body may simply need the extra hour of sleep. If no amount of sleep seems to be enough, you may have a sleep disorder, and you should consult your doctor.

Is there such a thing as too much sleep? Strictly speaking, no. Usually, people who spend a lot of time in bed are awake or lightly dozing, so they're not accumulating large amounts of deep sleep. But spending an excessive amount of time in bed may indicate a psychological problem. And someone with a need for sleep that interferes with his or her ability to function (say, 14 hours a day) requires medical treatment.

Once you've deprived yourself of sleep, do you try to "catch up" on your sleep? Perhaps because you only got four hours of sleep Sunday night, you promise yourself to hit the sack by 9:00 P.M. Monday night. That will give you 11 hours of sleep, which is surely enough to balance the scales, right? While this strategy may help improve daytime sleepiness on Tuesday somewhat, it tends to throw off your body clock (described in Remedy 24).

The best strategy is to schedule a regular sleep period and stick to it. The impact of insufficient sleep is too great for you to be nonchalant about it. Pay attention to the signals your body sends you. It will tell you how much sleep you need.

SET YOUR VCR.

It's 11:30 P.M. and you're ready to turn in for the night. The local news is just ending, and you reach for the remote control to turn off the television. But wait. Just before you hit the Off button, a commercial for the late movie comes on. *Night of the Living Dead*—your favorite movie—will be shown in its entirety, without commercial interruption.

You quickly weigh the options: either stay up to watch the movie and be very sleepy at work tomorrow, or wait another six months until the movie airs again. Choosing to ignore the consequences, you run to the kitchen, grab a bag of popcorn, and settle in to watch the movie. At 1:30 A.M. the last of the monsters is done in, and you go to sleep. Unfortunately, you wake up the next morning feeling like one of the zombies in the movie and stumble through the day.

Twenty years ago, choices in this situation were limited; you could either watch the movie or not. But the invention of the videocassette recorder has changed all of that. Now we can record our favorite television shows and watch them at our convenience.

Yet many people fail to use the VCR to its full potential.

If you have a VCR, use it. Whether you are constantly staying up past your bedtime to catch a late movie, a ball game, or reruns of *Gilligan's Island,* the VCR is invaluable. To those of you who don't know how to program your VCR, we have one word: Learn. (Hint: Ask someone younger than you for help. Young people between the ages of 8 and 16 are your best bet. They seem to have been born with the ability to understand electronic equipment.) To tape a program that starts at your bedtime, you don't even have to set the timer. (Look for the record button, usually marked REC, and push it. The machine will stop recording when it runs out of tape.)

If you find yourself frequently up late to watch television and you don't own a VCR, consider buying one. The newer models are inexpensive and easy to use. The modest cost will be repaid by your improved sleep. And the program you wanted to see will be there the next evening or on the weekend when you can enjoy it fully.

NAP SPARINGLY.

If you're tired during the day and the opportunity arises, you'll probably want to nap. Napping can help if you're exhausted or stressed out. The better rested you are, the better you'll be able to function. A short snooze can often restore much-needed energy.

However, too much napping may end up doing more harm than good. During a long nap you might reach the deep stages of sleep from which it is difficult to fully recover. You could easily wake up cranky and more tired than when you started. Worse still, too much sleep during the day will keep you up at night.

Have you ever taken a nap in an attempt to "store up" sleep for later? Perhaps you knew you would be out very late and you wanted to make sure you could stay awake. This strategy may help to keep you awake at night, but it may also disrupt your sleep rhythm.

If you must nap, keep it short. A 15- or 20-minute nap will help you feel refreshed without throwing off your body's sleep rhythm or causing insomnia at night.

DON'T SLEEP LATE ON WEEKENDS.

It's Sunday night. 11:00 P.M. You have to be up for work Monday morning at 6:00, and you desperately need sleep after a long weekend of late nights out. But your body refuses to co-operate. You lie in bed, tossing and turning, with each passing minute becoming more anxious about how you will survive the next day without any sleep. You begin to think your desire for sleep is the only dream you're likely to have this night. Finally, at a little past 3:00 A.M., sleep finally comes. Moments later (or so it seems) the alarm clock goes off. Morning has arrived much, much too soon.

Sunday night insomnia has probably affected everyone at one time or another. This kind of insomnia is caused by the resetting of your body's internal clocks when you shift to a later bedtime on Friday and Saturday night. On midnight Sunday, your body thinks the time is closer to 9:00 P.M. and time to start another party! It's no surprise then that sleep comes only with great difficulty.

Unfortunately, you cannot entirely avoid Sunday night insomnia unless you are willing to make changes in your lifestyle. But you can reduce the effects of late-night weekends.

- Be reasonable about late hours. Staying up a few hours past your weekday bedtime should cause only minor problems, but avoid staying up until 4:00 or 5:00 A.M. or pulling "all-nighters."

- Even if you are out late, try to get up at a time close to your usual time of waking. Do not sleep more than two hours beyond the time you usually wake up or it will be difficult to recover before the work week begins.

- Forget about making up for lost sleep with long afternoon naps. You are much better off enduring a small amount of sleepiness on the weekends than suffering through an entire week with severe sleepiness and insomnia.

LEAVE JET LAG BEHIND.

Several methods have been devised for preventing jet lag. There's even one that involves an elaborate system of changes in diet. The only problem with these methods is they don't work. The only sure method for combating jet lag is to begin adjusting your own biological clocks before leaving for your destination. This approach is sometimes cumbersome because it means altering your sleep-wake schedule. But it definitely works. A trip from New York to London provides an example of this technique.

Suppose your usual New York bedtime is midnight and your usual waking time is 7:00 A.M. When you go to bed at midnight, it is already 5:00 A.M. in merry old England. Your biological clocks are, therefore, five hours behind local time in London. But what if you went to bed early one night, say at 11:00 P.M.? Your body clocks would shift one hour from your habitual bedtime. But rather than 5:00 A.M. London time, you are now going to sleep at 4:00 A.M. London time—one hour closer to your regular New York bedtime of midnight. The idea is that as you retire progressively earlier, your body clocks move closer to London time. If you went to bed at 9:00 P.M., that would be 2:00 A.M. London time—a mere two hours from your usual midnight bedtime in New York.

How do you apply this idea in a real life situation? Imagine it is July 2 and you are going overseas July 8 on a two-week tour of English and Scottish castles. At the moment, your body clocks are five hours behind London time. So you don't waste a moment of your trip, over the next week you gradually adjust these internal clocks so they are closer to local time in London. You do this by going to bed a little earlier each day from July 2 until you depart so that on the night of July 7, you go to bed at 9:00 P.M. When you get to London, your body clock will be only two hours different from local time, an adjustment that can be made quickly and with few of the effects of jet lag.

Prior to your return from England you follow the same process, only this time in reverse. Instead of going to bed 30 minutes earlier each night, you go to bed one hour later. Note the shift is faster when travel is from London (East) to the United States (West) rather than from West to East. This is a general rule for travel across time zones: Adapting to time changes is easier and faster with westerly travel than easterly travel.

Unfortunately, for travel across more than five or six time zones, this process becomes unwieldy. In the worst case, a crossing of exactly 12 time zones, it is usually impossible to come close to fully shifting your body clocks. In this case, you would shift as much as practical prior to departure. When you arrive at your destination, immediately begin operating on local time; that is, sleep at night and be up and active during the day. While you will probably experience some of the symptoms of jet lag for at least several days, you will have reduced the severity of the problem.

If jet lag hits you particularly hard, you may wish to consult a sleep specialist who can provide advice specific to your situation. Such counseling is not inexpensive, but when you consider the amount you have invested in your vacation or that millions of dollars may hinge on the outcome of overseas business negotiations, such assistance may prove a wise investment.

USE YOUR BED FOR SLEEP AND SEX ONLY.

Most of us think of our bed as a place mainly for sleeping. But it's also likely most of us use it for more than just sleep. We may watch television, talk on the telephone, eat, read, or play cards. Children often find the bed makes an excellent trampoline.

To get the best sleep, however, you should not perform any of these activities in bed. When you do, the bed and bedroom become associated with activities other than sleep, which makes sleep more difficult. Your body can become conditioned to respond to the bed and the bedroom by becoming alert rather than drowsy.

Some people actually work in bed. While this practice may shorten your commute, it can seriously disrupt your sleep. When you work in bed, all of the associated stress becomes related to the bed and bedroom. Just getting into bed at night may then cause your heart rate to increase, your muscles to tighten, and your brain to become active. Whether you consciously realize it, the sheets, blankets, and pillows are now associated with your job, and their very sight and smell will cause thoughts of work to flood your mind as you try to fall asleep.

For these same reasons, you should not read or watch television in bed. Your body will take getting into bed as a signal for those activities and react accordingly. Eating in bed is definitely a bad idea. You don't want your stomach to start growling every time you pull back the covers! Also, crumbs in bed are not especially comfortable.

The single exception to this rule involves sex. Sexual activity in bed will not disturb sleep. In fact, sleep usually follows quickly and easily. Sex with a partner or masturbation can be very relaxing and promote a peaceful and restful night. So, as another way to get a good night's rest, reserve the bed for sleep and sex only.

CAN'T SLEEP? GET OUT OF BED.

Do you have nights when, instead of sleeping, you toss, turn, squirm, and fidget? Contrary to common belief, the solution is not to stay in bed, hoping sleep will come. Consider this: If you spend a quarter of each night squirming under your sheets, the bedroom will become a very unpleasant place for you. You will associate your room and your bed with feeling frustrated, uncomfortable, and unhappy. When you walk into your room, you'll immediately begin to worry about how long it will take you to fall asleep. Consequently, it will take you longer.

If you can't sleep, don't stay in bed. Let your body associate any feelings of wakefulness with some other part of your home. Go to the kitchen for a drink of water. Read. Sew. Draw. Examine the operating instructions to your VCR. Anything will do—as long as it's relaxing and doesn't require intense concentration. Gradually, you'll become tired and bored. Usually, within 15 to 20 minutes your body will be ready for you to try to sleep again.

LIMIT THE LIGHT.

Although it might seem ridiculously obvious, it is important to eliminate light from the bedroom at night. If a light shines into your room at night, take steps to eliminate it. Purchase shades or curtains, but make sure they are not translucent. Eye shades are an inexpensive option and are also useful when traveling.

If you sleep with a nightlight, make sure it is dim enough that you cannot sense it when you shut your eyes. If you usually use the bathroom at night, leave a night-light on in the bathroom so you don't have to turn on any lights. Exposing yourself to bright light in the middle of the night may needlessly increase the time it takes to return to sleep.

USE A TIMER.

Imagine you are in bed at night, drifting off as Ted Koppel grills a recently indicted politician, when suddenly . . .

RATATATAT! You are roused from sleep by the staccato of semiautomatic gunfire. No, your home is not under attack; but *Nightline* is over, and a 1930's gangster movie has taken its place. You reach for the remote control, turn off the television, and wearily return to sleep.

This scene is repeated thousands of time every night in homes across the country. Many people enjoy falling asleep with the TV or radio playing, and many others have difficulty getting to sleep without the background noise. However, the soft music or quiet chatter that puts you to sleep can disturb sleep later on.

Even though you may feel your sleep is sound and restful when the television or radio plays through the night, the noise or light actually causes small arousals and awakenings. Most people are unaware of these awakenings—but they may feel the effects the next day. Sleep specialists estimate most of us experience about 20 of these awakenings each night. If you sleep with the radio or TV on, you may awaken even more than that. Of course, even if you can sleep through the usual late-night fare of shootouts, car chases, and sitcom repeats, you would probably spring to attention when the national anthem is played. And who hasn't trudged out of bed at 4:00 A.M. to turn off the TV test pattern?

The best answer is to leave the TV or radio off. If you usually have the TV on at bedtime, try several nights with the room quiet. Sleep may come with surprising ease. If you really need the sound to fall asleep, use a timer to turn it off or purchase a radio with a "Sleep" function. Another option is to generate a noise that will not cause frequent awakenings; see Remedy 37 for tips on how to do this.

Having the late show on while you sleep may make for some pretty interesting dreams, but the peace and quiet you'll have with the TV or radio off will promote uninterrupted sleep and help leave you refreshed the next day.

MOVING? CHECK OUT THE NEIGHBORHOOD.

Obviously, many factors determine where we live. But if you can control your environment at all, you should keep your sleep needs in mind. Don't underestimate the stress and irritation a noisy neighborhood can cause.

Investigate possible sources of noise when you are looking for a new house or apartment. Here are a few suggestions:

- Ask other tenants or home owners whether the neighbors are considerate about keeping noise to a minimum.

- Look at the area immediately around the house or apartment building. Does the house next door have ten cars parked in the driveway and street? That may be a sign that people come and go frequently. How close is the building next door? If your neighbors have balconies or back porches, how close are they to your bedroom window? In warm weather, will a late-night barbecue disturb your sleep? Does the neighbor's dog bark every time someone walks by?

- Don't overlook certain features of an apartment. Check the thickness of the walls.
Can you hear the television of the tenants
next door? (Visit the apartment during the
day and at night to check the noise level in
the building.) Those newly polished wood
floors may be beautiful, but do they mean
you will then hear every step your upstairs
neighbor takes? If the apartment has
steam radiators, can you live with the
banging and hissing they produce? Is the
apartment directly over the garage or main
entryway?

- Ask about the other tenants. How many people live upstairs? Are seven people sharing a
one bedroom apartment? Or, does the sweet
young couple living there have newborn
twins or young children who love to stomp?
Is the young man across the hall a bass
player in a rock band who practices at home?
Ask, too, about the schedules of other tenants in an apartment building. Does the
woman upstairs use her NordicTrack at 5:00
A.M. before she leaves for work?

- Walk around the neighborhood in the daytime, the evening, and at night. That quaint
tavern may be charming in the day but a

source of loud conversation (or worse) at night. Being near a school is terrific for the children, but get too close and the marching band's practices could disturb an afternoon nap for a night shift worker. The park across the street is lovely, but is it a popular gathering spot at all hours? Are you near a fire station?

- Check out the traffic patterns in the area. The bus stop near your front door may seem very convenient, until you realize your whole apartment shakes each time a bus starts and stops there on its 24-hour route. The same may be true if the home is located along a truck route. You may be miles from the local airport, but take-off and landing patterns may be right over your house.

Be alert that high prices and fancy addresses are no guarantee of peace and quiet. (If noise around your current home is a problem, try to generate some noise of your own to mask the sound. See Remedy 37 for tips on how to do this.) Obviously, you cannot eliminate all the noise or find a place that meets all your noise-related criteria, but you should at least think about whether your new home will be a place you can get some rest.

GENERATE SOME NOISE!

Our sleeping environments are rarely sound-free. There may be trains roaring by, planes overhead, people yelling in the street, or birds chirping and calling in the early morning. The best solution, of course, is to eliminate the noise. But airports, highways, 24-hour diners, our neighbors, and the local animal population are not likely to move so we may sleep better. So rather than eliminate the cause of nighttime noise pollution, mask the noise with a white noise generator.

White noise generators are sound-producing devices. With one push of a button they make a soft, whooshing noise that drowns out the sudden and unpredictable noises that can disturb sleep. The noise is easy to get used to and rarely causes any disturbance by itself—the sound is actually quite soothing. More sophisticated models can produce the sounds of rain, wind, or the sea shore.

Unlike the television or a radio, the noise produced by a white noise generator does not cause awakenings because there are no volume changes and the sound itself is unchanging. Also, because the noise from the generator contains many different frequencies, it literally keeps our ear busy and focused on these steady, uninteresting, but complex sounds.

You can purchase white noise generators at many large department stores, in specialty shops, and through mail-order catalogs. They're affordable, ranging in price from $50 to $150, and simple to use. Because a generator is about the size of an alarm clock, you can position it at the head of the bed or the foot, on a nightstand or the floor, or anywhere the sound benefits you the most.

In the summer months, you can substitute a ceiling fan, quiet floor or window fan, or room air conditioner for a white noise generator.

38

HUMIDIFY YOUR HOME.

You're hot and your throat is parched. Each swallow is agonizingly difficult. Your skin is dry and cracked, and your eyes are burning. All you can think of is a tall, cool glass of water.

Where is this scene from? The Sahara Desert? Death Valley? The planet Venus? No, this is the typical environment in a North American home in winter, where the artificial heat that keeps us warm also dries out the air we breathe.

Although most of us prefer a temperature of 68 degrees or higher in the winter, we may pay a price for all that warmth. Heating systems not only warm the surrounding air, but they remove a lot of moisture from the air as well. As you breathe the hot, dry air, water is also removed from your breathing passages. Too much moisture loss in the airway can lead to throat or nasal discomfort or even upper airway infection. (Influenza viruses thrive in an atmosphere of low humidity.) And if you've ever tried to sleep with a cold or the flu caused by such an infection, you know it's very difficult to get a good night's rest. In addition, many people awaken several or more times in a night to get a glass of water to soothe their dry, parched throats, which also disturbs sleep.

Fortunately, there is a simple and inexpensive solution to the dry air caused by indoor heating: a room humidifier. A humidifier adds moisture to the air and counters the effects of dry, indoor heat. Increased humidity will not only make sleep easier but provide a generally more comfortable and healthful environment. Humidifying your home helps prevent the spread of viruses, and it eases some of your discomfort if you have a respiratory infection. Just be sure to clean the unit frequently to combat the growth of bacteria and replace any filters according to the manufacturer's instructions.

You can also keep a pot of water on low boil on the stove or place a pot of water on a radiator to add moisture to the air.

Incidentally, most humidifiers also act as white noise generators. See Remedy 37 for more information on these valuable sleep tools.

FIND THE RIGHT TEMPERATURE.

Room temperature can profoundly impact sleep quality. What Goldilocks learned of porridge is also true of sleep: Neither too hot nor too cold is very good. Many people accept extreme temperatures as a fact of life or consider the expense of temperature control too great and allow their sleep to suffer as a result. Actually, it is possible to cope with almost any temperature, high or low, without taking out a second mortgage on the house.

When summer heat is a problem, consider buying an air conditioner for the bedroom. Yes, they can be expensive to purchase, install, and run, but an air conditioner keeps you cool and blocks out street noise. In the long run, a comfortable bedroom may be well worth the price. Many modern units are highly energy efficient, and the cost of using one may be less than you think. Ceiling and window fans can be effective as well. As another bonus, some of these devices generate white noise. See Remedy 37 for information on the value of white noise generators in getting a good night's sleep.

Cold weather seems relatively easy to deal with. Certainly, you could just crank up the heat. Although effective, this simple solution can be quite costly. And if you live in an older building with steam radiators, you may not have control over the heat. Try wearing flannel or other warm nightclothes, placing flannel sheets on the bed, and piling on layers of blankets. These products will provide adequate warmth even in the coldest climes at a minimal cost.

But what if your husband prefers a nice, warm bedroom when you are (or so he claims) descended from a race of penguins? Separate bedrooms are one possibility, though this solution is hardly conducive to marital bliss. The alternatives usually involve a nightly battle over the window or the air conditioner or heater controls. It is not unheard of for one spouse to open a window several times a night, only to have the other spouse close it each time. Such disagreement is not only bad for sleep but can be stressful for the relationship. Compromise on room temperature is always possible, but this might mean no one is comfortable at night. A better solution is to ensure both of you are as comfortable as possible.

Here are a few tips to follow when you and your bed partner have widely varying internal thermostats.

- Dress for the temperature you prefer, not for the temperature outside. This generally means you and your spouse will have to dress very differently. In the winter while your husband is wearing flannel pajamas, you may be dressed in a light nightgown or T-shirt.

- Use layers of blankets. A sheet, a light cotton blanket, a wool blanket, and a thick comforter are a good complete set for your bed. You may want to purchase twin sizes, even for larger beds, so you each have your own set of blankets. A number of blankets ensures that you and your bed partner can select the amount of "coverage" you want. Add flannel sheets to this equation and you can be sure your bed partner stays warm. Then while he is nestled between the flannel sheets and four blankets, you can be comfortable with just a sheet and a light blanket. (And if your bed partner is warm and cozy beneath his covers, he may not mind so much that you must have the window open.) Note, though, that not all blankets are equal. Some fabrics tend to "breathe" better, meaning they keep you warm but allow perspiration to escape through the fabric, so you stay dry and comfortable and don't get overheated.

- Consider purchasing an electric blanket with dual heating elements. With this arrangement, both partners have their own thermostat and can regulate the temperature without causing the other any discomfort. The cost is modest and you get lots of heat. The risk of fire has been virtually eliminated with the newer models.

Another hint for all you frosty folk with a warm-blooded bed partner: Make good use of the burning ember next to you. In other words, people who are usually warm generate a lot of heat. So sidle up a little closer, and let the heat from your bed partner help keep you warm.

40

CHOOSE THE RIGHT MATTRESS.

We spend about one third of our lives asleep, and most of this time is spent lying on a mattress. Despite the amount of time we spend in bed, many of us ignore our mattress until the springs start poking us through the mattress pad. But a mattress has a lot to do with the quality of our sleep and, therefore, a lot to do with how we feel during the day. So give some thought and attention to the type of mattress you use to ensure a good night's sleep and a well-rested feeling the following day.

When selecting a mattress, you need to make decisions about the degree of firmness, the type of mattress (and bed), and the size you prefer.

Firmness

Don't assume soft and fluffy is best. Poor support can lead to muscle stiffness as well as neck and back pain. Make sure your mattress isn't too soft and doesn't contain bumps, valleys, or depressions.

Of course, too stiff isn't great either. A mattress that is too hard can put pressure on the shoulders and hips. The ideal surface is gently supportive and firm, not rock hard or squishy.

Keep in mind that mattresses don't last forever. Gradually, over time, they lose their firmness and support. Once your mattress has developed lumps and sags, it is definitely time to replace it.

Type

Along with a wide variety of comfort needs comes a wide variety of mattress and bed types. What are your options? The most common type of bedding is the box spring mattress. These mattresses contain inner steel coils of various thicknesses and configurations, resulting in different degrees of firmness. Test several to find the one that suits you best. Another common type of bedding is the polyurethane foam mattress. Different thicknesses provide for a wide variety of support and comfort.

Water beds are very popular, but you need to be careful when purchasing a water bed or you risk sinking in a sea of troubles. Water beds are expensive, require 200 gallons of water, take up lots of space, and sometimes leak. A heater is usually necessary. But if you're willing to spend the money, you can get a high-quality water bed. Just make sure the water chamber is deep and properly filled and the manufacturer has a good reputation.

Be sure to sample somebody else's water bed before buying your own. Floating around all night might seem like a lot of fun, but the fantasy of a water bed may be better than the reality. The constant wavelike motion doesn't work for everyone. Incidentally, if you want a water bed, but your bed partner gets seasick going to the beach, a water bed with multiple chambers may be a good compromise. A chambered water bed holds the water in multiple, independent units, usually cylinders. This design minimizes sloshing because water is restricted to a single cylinder.

Electrically controlled beds are another possibility. Certainly, it's convenient to raise and lower the bed at the touch of a button. But these beds are very expensive for general use. If you have a medical reason for needing one, your insurance may help cover the cost.

Size

Along with deciding what kind of mattress you want, you need to figure out what size. As a rule, bigger is better. You don't want to fight for space every night or get kicked, elbowed, or shoved on a regular basis. A healthy sleeper moves around from 15 to 30 times during the night, and cramped conditions can make sleeping awkward, uncomfortable, and altogether frustrating. Also, as you and your bed partner get older, your sleep will become more restless and you may require extra room in bed. Get the largest mattress that fits in your bedroom and your budget.

You spend about eight hours each day in bed, and the quality of your sleep determines how you feel the rest of the day. So think about the type of mattress you want and shop carefully. Sample a variety of mattresses. The right mattress will go a long way toward ensuring peaceful nights of uninterrupted sleep.

CHOOSE PILLOWS WITH CARE.

Like the choice of a mattress, the choice of a pillow is a very personal matter. Although some people can sleep with their head on a rock, most of us are very particular about the type of pillows we use. Your choice of pillows and how you position them have a lot to do with the quality of your sleep.

The majority of people use a single pillow, but it certainly is all right to use more than one. If you prefer to have your head elevated, a wedge-shaped pillow might suit you. But be careful to identify the reason you need to elevate your head. For example, if you experience shortness of breath when you sleep flat or with a single pillow, let your doctor know. This symptom could indicate a serious medical problem. Don't pile up the pillows as a way to ease the discomfort of heartburn. Elevate the bed instead (see Remedy 7 for more information).

If your nose starts to run and you sneeze every time your head touches the pillow, you may be allergic to your pillow. Many pillows are filled with goose down or other natural materials that are common allergens. Try a pillow made with foam or another synthetic material to solve the problem.

"Orthopedic pillows" can help relieve pain and stiffness from injuries to the neck or upper back. They are usually made of a special foam and are often recognizable by their shape. Orthopaedic pillows are more expensive than conventional pillows, but medical insurance may cover their purchase if your doctor prescribes them. You can purchase these pillows at a surgical supply store.

Also available are pillows designed to reduce or eliminate snoring. Despite the rather optimistic claims about these pillows, they are rarely effective. For a major snoring problem, consult a sleep specialist (see Remedy 5).

Most important, find a pillow that makes you comfortable. Just because your Aunt Griselda uses pillows made with hair from the East African two-humped camel doesn't mean you should. Try a variety of types and stick with the one that provides you with the best night of sleep.

MOVE ROVER OVER—AND FLUFFY, TOO!

In the American household, pets are considered part of the family. Deference to our dogs, cats, and other pets may extend to sleeping arrangements. A favored pet may stake claim to the bed, perhaps even trying to take your place on the bed.

Some pets are leaners—in other words, they like to put their head, paw, or entire body on some part of your body. When that becomes annoying, you move over—only to have your pet follow you, leaning once again. Eventually, you find you've shifted nearly off the bed, and your pet has the best spot on the bed—yours. Ring any bells?

Although you might think otherwise, the bed may not really be big enough for you and your pet. Animals can move around at night just as people do. In the same way a bed partner's movements arouse you from sleep, so does movement of your dog or cat. When the bed is occupied by another person as well as one or more pets, the net result can be markedly fragmented sleep. If the pet is large or bed space limited, then the maneuvering for room can make sleep downright uncomfortable. Battling a slobbering St. Bernard who insists your pillow is his favorite resting place will not result in a good night's sleep.

Then there are pets that wake their owners just for company. (Ever awoken to find one of your pet's favorite toys on your pillow?)

If any of these scenarios sound familiar, it's time to bar your pets from your bed. If you must, keep the door to your bedroom closed when you sleep. Moving your pet from the bed may be painful. You might even feel this is an act of betrayal. In truth, your pet will not love you less, but you will live together in greater peace and comfort.

An issue that involves dog owners is the need to walk the dog. Dogs usually need to go out in the morning and, unfortunately, often before you would like to get out of bed. Depending upon your housing arrangements, you can solve this problem several ways.

- If you have a fenced yard, consider using a small door through which your dog can come and go as it pleases.

- Train your dog to go outside at a later time. Often a dog can wait to go out but has simply established a habit of waking early.

- Put off Rover's late night walk till the last possible minute. This may keep him sleeping a little later in the morning.

Even if your pet doesn't need to go out in the morning, he may wake you when he's hungry, particularly if you usually feed your pet first thing in the morning. Many pet owners will attest to the fact that it's very difficult to catch even just one extra hour of sleep on the weekend if they have a pet that's accustomed to eating at 6:00 A.M. Again, you can keep the door to the bedroom closed so Rover and Fluffy don't wake you with nudges and whimpers. But hungry pets can be very persistent, so the scratching or whining at the bedroom door will probably keep you from sleeping. For the sake of both of you, consider shifting your pet's meal times. After a brief, though sometimes difficult, transition period, your pet may benefit from having a well-rested friend.

LEARN DOROTHY'S LESSON: THERE'S NO PLACE LIKE HOME.

When speaking of sleep, one could easily quote Dorothy from *The Wizard of Oz:* There is no place like home. Even in lavish surroundings in four star hotels, you usually don't sleep as well as you do in your own bed.

The poor sleep that often occurs in a strange environment is known as *the first night effect*. This name is appropriate because sleep often improves considerably after as little as one night away from home.

One trick to getting sound sleep when away from home is to make the environment seem more familiar and homelike. One simple way to do this is to bring along some objects from home. Bring your own pillow, for example. A stuffed animal (don't be embarrassed!) or other reminder of your own bed also makes you more comfortable and helps you sleep.

When you're away from home, try to follow your usual routine in the hour before bed. If you read before bed, bring along a book or grab the local newspaper. If you watch a particular television program, do the same. Give your body all its usual clues bedtime is approaching.

If, on the other hand, you find you sleep better away from home, you should try to determine why. What did the new sleep environment have that your bedroom at home did not? No pets? Better pillows? A firmer mattress? A quieter environment? Distance from life's problems?

These advantages may contribute to better sleep. But it's more likely that individuals who sleep better away from home have a *psychophysiologic insomnia.* In simpler terms, they don't sleep well at home because something makes them associate their home sleep environment with wakefulness. This association does not exist in the new environment, so they sleep better. If you sleep better when you're away, consider that stress at home or at work may block restful sleep at home.

SET LIMITS FOR CHILDREN.

Probably no parent has been spared a child's bedtime request to stay up "just five more minutes." The number of excuses children give for staying up later are almost beyond counting: "I'm hungry/thirsty . . . I need to go to the bathroom . . . I want to watch television/hear another story . . . There are monsters in my room . . ." and on and on *ad infinitum.*

When the attempts to stay up past bedtime are infrequent or related to special occasions, they do not indicate a real problem. Allowing your child a rare night up past his or her regular bedtime is generally harmless. However, when a child repeatedly puts up a fight at bedtime, something must be done. Children require more sleep than adults—as much as 10 to 12 hours—and an earlier bedtime is essential to their physical and mental wellbeing.

Most often, persistent difficulty in getting a child to bed comes from not having established comforting and regular bedtime routines. Some parents are cavalier when a child first resists bedtime and do not respond until the situation becomes a real problem. Figure out a good bedtime for your child, and make settling him or her in at that time a priority. When a child derives comfort and pleasure from a nightly routine, he or she is much less inclined to struggle when bedtime nears.

Less often, an underlying conflict needs to be resolved. Sometimes the struggle for bedtime is a purposeful challenge to parental authority. At other times, a child has carried some underlying fear—for example, of abandonment—over from the daytime. A discussion with your child may reveal the problem and greatly assist in finding a solution. Ask about your child's fears, worries, and thoughts, and listen carefully to the response. Was she upset about your long vacation without her? How are things with the baby-sitter? With friends? Is he afraid of something or someone? How is school? Discussions with teachers can also be helpful.

At any age, children can experience stress and depression. Altered sleep patterns may be one of the few signs that parents can detect. Family illness, family conflicts, separations, and school problems can cause sleep problems. Teenagers inevitably face problems with self-confidence, self-esteem, sexual identity, and sexual orientation. Sleep problems, therefore, might be the tip of the iceberg of problems that require discussions among parents and children or even professional help. Talk with your child's doctor, a sleep center, or other pediatric specialists for guidance on helping your child with any problems that impact sleep. Whatever you do, avoid intense discussions just before bedtime. A quiet, comforting, and loving bedtime routine can only be helpful.

If your children are watched by a relative, baby-sitter, or other caretaker, their bedtime routines should not change. Children feel comforted by consistency from night to night and person to person. When parents are separated or divorced, a parent should not curry favor with the children by allowing a later bedtime.

While most children require 10 to 12 hours of sleep, sleep needs can vary. Parents should not simply go by the book and insist their child sleep 12 hours when, for that child, nine hours is enough. Sleep needs can change as well. A child who was once an 11-hour sleeper may require only nine hours at age seven or eight. Insisting the child go to bed at 7:00 when he or she will not fall asleep until 9:00

just creates problems. Be sensitive to the child's needs and help him or her settle on a routine that fulfills those needs.

Letting children stay up late because it is convenient for the parents usually leads to inconvenience down the road. A child who habitually goes to bed late and sleeps late may allow parents to sleep late, too. But any benefit to parents will be short-lived and will ultimately backfire. The night-owl child haunts parents late at night then tortures them in the morning when they try to get the child up.

Incidentally, don't let schoolchildren sleep late on weekends. The reasons described in Remedy 30 apply to children, too. If a child is scheduled to begin school for the first time or to return after a summer off, be sure to establish an early bedtime a good week before school starts. You may want to move your child's bedtime earlier and earlier, gradually over a week.

READ OR SING TO CHILDREN AT BEDTIME.

Most parents recognize the importance of the period just before bedtime. They engage in a special ritual that helps secure the bond with their child, provide a sense a security, and help the child get to sleep. This important activity is usually referred to as "tucking the child in."

Tucking a child into bed is an art, not a science. There are no rules that hold in every case and at every bedtime. Happily, word and song have a sleep-inducing effect that almost all children respond to.

Reading to your child often helps induce sleep. Most children repeatedly ask for one or two favorite books at bedtime. Reserve these books for reading at night, keeping them on the shelf during the day. The idea is to associate a particular story with bedtime, so its mere mention causes drowsiness. When you read, it is all right to reflect some of the story's emotion, but keep your voice low and your tone soft.

Music is another means to soothe a rambunctious child at bedtime. Singing a lullaby is a wonderful method to put a child to sleep and establish a parent-child bond. Of course, if you think your singing sounds more like beetles than the Beatles, a commercial tape of lullabies does just fine. Some stuffed animals and dolls play lullabies; these toys can also double as transitional objects to help children gain some independence (see Remedy 47).

Whatever method of tucking in you choose, remember the most important component is your presence. At this time of day, childhood fears of the dark, abandonment, and even death become most pronounced. Therefore, bedtime is a perfect opportunity to dispel these fears and communicate feelings of love. It may also be the only time of day when parent and child can interact without the distractions common at other hours. This quiet time allows for the development of a closeness that occurs only rarely during the daylight hours.

SWITCH SLEEP POSITIONS TO HELP PREVENT SIDS.

Every year, 6,000 infants in the United States die as a result of the terrifying yet unexplained phenomenon *sudden infant death syndrome,* or SIDS. Babies who seemed perfectly normal and healthy are found lifeless in their cribs. Despite intensive research and investigation, these deaths remain unexplained. SIDS remains the second-leading cause of death among children younger than one year old. A single cause for SIDS has not been found, and most cases still have no explanation. However, new studies indicate there is a way to prevent at least some of these tragic deaths.

For years, doctors have been telling parents to put their children to bed on their stomachs. But because of the new studies, doctors now advise that infants be placed on their backs or sides to sleep. How does sleeping position relate to SIDS? When a child sleeps face down, the carbon dioxide he or she exhales can be trapped in the bedding or pillow. Experts believe if an infant then inhales too much of this trapped carbon dioxide, cessation in breathing can occur, which may result in death.

The soft pillows, blankets, and mattresses commonly used in infants' bedding seem to make this occurrence more likely. For this reason, experts recommend firm bedding for an infant younger than age one.

New products are available to help the infant stay on his or her back or side. Your pediatrician can help determine if these products are right for your child. Some infants may need to use an electronic monitor with an alarm. Again, your child's doctor is the best source for information.

Breast-feeding and good prenatal care also appear to reduce the chance SIDS will occur. Also avoid keeping the infant's room too warm, and do not smoke around your infant. Following these guidelines helps ensure your infant sleeps safely and soundly. And knowing your infant is protected by these measures should help you sleep better as well.

GIVE TODDLERS A TRANSITIONAL OBJECT.

Every adult certainly knows it: Growing up is tough. At each stage of development—infant, toddler, young child, adolescent—there are particular challenges to meet and obstacles to overcome—even where sleep is concerned. When it comes to sleep, one of the most difficult periods involves the toddler stage. At this point, a child is generally expected to sleep through the night without waking the parents. Unfortunately, this is not always the case.

To help sleep at this stage, you can give your child a special helper called a *transitional object*. The name comes from the object's use during the transition period from the child's total dependence to partial independence. The transitional object, usually a blanket or stuffed animal, eases the way for a child to separate from his or her parents, especially (in most cases) the mother. Because the object is soft and fluffy, it can convey a sense of physical warmth and closeness. Because it is always there, it can convey a sense of permanence and stability. These comforts are especially important at night-time when the child is falling asleep or awakes during the night.

As a rule, a child takes the object wherever he or she goes. It is much more than just another toy. The transitional object is uniquely important in providing comfort and security. The child will develop an attachment to it which compares to nothing else. When you wash it, for example, don't be surprised if your son or daughter sits in front of the dryer waiting for the final cycle to finish.

Although the value of the transitional object goes beyond helping sleep, that is one of its most important functions. Your child must learn to fall asleep without your physical presence. Also, when children awake in the night, they must learn to return to sleep without calling for you each time. The transitional object helps provide both you and your child with an uninterrupted night of sleep.

TAKE KIDS FOR A RIDE.

The problem of the child who resists sleep is not new. Entire books have been written on the subject. Yet even many young children who are normally good sleepers resist sleep every once in a while.

If your child can't or won't sleep, tell him or her you're going to go for a short drive. Then drive around the block a few times. More often than not, your child will quickly fall asleep.

This may not be the most scientific method; it has never been formally studied in the laboratory, and no research data exist. Nevertheless, it has been field tested by the ultimate authorities: parents with cranky children. The technique usually works with children up to about age six and provides an easy solution for the child who occasionally has difficulty falling asleep. Remedy 44 describes some alternative methods.

If your child repeatedly can't or won't sleep, ask your child's doctor for help.

LEAD SLEEPWALKERS BACK TO BED.

Sleepwalking in children is extremely common because their sleep is so deep. When something happens to arouse them in the night, the part of the brain responsible for waking them cannot easily overcome the part responsible for sleep. The result is a state in which the child is partly awake and partly asleep.

Children sleepwalk with their eyes open and can see objects around them. Nevertheless, they may misinterpret what they see. A window may appear to be a door and the child could attempt to climb out. While children are usually able to go up and down stairs while sleepwalking, they may do so clumsily, and a fall could result. It is, therefore, important to protect a child known to sleepwalk by locking windows, barricading stairways, and removing hazardous objects from their immediate vicinity.

Children who walk in their sleep generally do not need medical attention. When sleepwalking occurs only occasionally and does not involve vigorous behaviors, it is not considered abnormal. Most children outgrow the problem by early adolescence. Parents need only know how to handle sleepwalking episodes when they do occur.

Contrary to popular belief, waking a sleepwalking child is not dangerous. However, a child who awakens suddenly in strange surroundings may become frightened and confused. Since it is usually unnecessary to wake the child, let the sleepwalking continue. Most times, you will be able to gently take your child by the hand and lead him or her back to bed. Be persistent but not forceful or confrontational. The child will probably have no memory of the episode in the morning. Proper handling of the sleepwalking episode ensures you and your child get the good night's sleep both of you need.

As with sleepwalking, night terrors occur when the child is half awake and half asleep. The child screams loudly, disturbing any nearby sleepers. At times, the child may even dash out of bed screaming. The techniques for handling night terrors are the same as for sleepwalking: Protect the child from danger, carry on as few exchanges as possible, and guide the child back to bed. Do not ask the child to tell you why he or she is screaming or carrying on. The child doesn't know, often cannot answer at all, and will just get more agitated if you try to break him or her out of a half-sleep.

Parents may worry something is wrong with their child, and they may convey that worry to the child when they discuss the night's events the next day. Such events are most often a mysterious part of normal growth and development. It is important to recognize them as such so the child can be guided back to bed and the parent can return to sleep without worrying about what demons lurk within the child.

Sleepwalking and night terrors that persist into adolescence or young adulthood generally do not indicate psychological problems. Nevertheless, treatment with medication for older sleepwalkers is often helpful to restore normal sleep for the person and his or her roommates.

USE A NIGHT-LIGHT.

Overcoming fear of the dark and other childhood fears is an important part of growing up. A child may have worries related to family matters, such as fear of being abandoned following separation or divorce, or the child may simply be afraid of the dark. As a result of these fears, simple objects in the bedroom may take on new and ominous forms. A chair becomes a crouching intruder, the closet a home for demons and ghosts.

One way to help your child overcome these fears is to keep some light on in the child's bedroom at night. A night-light will not provide so much light that it disturbs your child's sleep, but it will provide enough to allay many of your child's fears. The chair will again be just a chair, and monsters will no longer be lurking in the closet. The light is comforting both for the illumination it provides and for its symbolism that a caretaker is very close by. And, as a practical matter, it makes it easier for the child to walk through the bedroom should he or she need to get up at night.

50 WAYS TO SLEEP BETTER